Diabetes
Log Book

Belongs to

Name: _____

Adress: _____

_____

Email: _____

Mobile Telephone: _____

Home Telephone: _____

Fax:

Diabetes Log Book

| Date: | | | | | M | T | W | T | F | S | S |

	Meal	Cal	Fat	Carbs	Total Sugar	Added Sugar	Protein	Fiber
BREAKFAST								
	Breakfast Totals							
	Blood Glucose Level	Befor:			Time:			
		After:			Time:			

	Meal	Cal	Fat	Carbs	Total Sugar	Added Sugar	Protein	Fiber
LUNCH								
	Lunch Totals							
	Blood Glucose Level	Befor:			Time:			
		After:			Time:			

	Meal	Cal	Fat	Carbs	Total Sugar	Added Sugar	Protein	Fiber
DINNER								
	Dinner Totals							
	Blood Glucose Level	Befor:			Time:			
		After:			Time:			

		Cal	Fat	Carbs	Total Sugar	Added Sugar	Protein	Fiber
SNACKS								
	Snack Totals							

Daily Totals							

Bedtime Blood Glucose Level		Time:	

Water	Sleep	Medication	Activity	Minutes	Notes

Diabetes Log Book

Date:						M T W T F S S		

	Meal	Cal	Fat	Carbs	Total Sugar	Added Sugar	Protein	Fiber
BREAKFAST								
	Breakfast Totals							
	Blood Glucose Level	Befor:				Time:		
		After:				Time:		

LUNCH								
	Lunch Totals							
	Blood Glucose Level	Befor:				Time:		
		After:				Time:		

DINNER								
	Dinner Totals							
	Blood Glucose Level	Befor:				Time:		
		After:				Time:		

SNACKS								
	Snack Totals							

Daily Totals							

Bedtime Blood Glucose Level		Time:	

Water	Sleep	Medication	Activity	Minutes	Notes

Diabetes Log Book

| Date: | | | | | | M T W T F S S | | | |

	Meal	Cal	Fat	Carbs	Total Sugar	Added Sugar	Protein	Fiber
BREAKFAST								
	Breakfast Totals							
	Blood Glucose Level	Befor:			Time:			
		After:			Time:			

	Meal	Cal	Fat	Carbs	Total Sugar	Added Sugar	Protein	Fiber
LUNCH								
	Lunch Totals							
	Blood Glucose Level	Befor:			Time:			
		After:			Time:			

	Meal	Cal	Fat	Carbs	Total Sugar	Added Sugar	Protein	Fiber
DINNER								
	DinnerTotals							
	Blood Glucose Level	Befor:			Time:			
		After:			Time:			

SNACKS								
	Snack Totals							

Daily Totals							

Bedtime Blood Glucose Level		Time:	

Water	Sleep	Medication	Activity	Minutes	Notes

Diabetes Log Book

Date:						M T W T F S S

	Meal	Cal	Fat	Carbs	Total Sugar	Added Sugar	Protein	Fiber
BREAKFAST								
	Breakfast Totals							
	Blood Glucose Level	Befor:				Time:		
		After:				Time:		

LUNCH								
	Lunch Totals							
	Blood Glucose Level	Befor:				Time:		
		After:				Time:		

DINNER								
	Dinner Totals							
	Blood Glucose Level	Befor:				Time:		
		After:				Time:		

SNACKS								
	Snack Totals							

Daily Totals							

Bedtime Blood Glucose Level		Time:	

Water	Sleep	Medication	Activity	Minutes	Notes

Diabetes Log Book

Date:					M T W T F S S			

	Meal	Cal	Fat	Carbs	Total Sugar	Added Sugar	Protein	Fiber
BREAKFAST								
	Breakfast Totals							
	Blood Glucose Level	Befor:				Time:		
		After:				Time:		

		Cal	Fat	Carbs	Total Sugar	Added Sugar	Protein	Fiber
LUNCH								
	Lunch Totals							
	Blood Glucose Level	Befor:				Time:		
		After:				Time:		

		Cal	Fat	Carbs	Total Sugar	Added Sugar	Protein	Fiber
DINNER								
	Dinner Totals							
	Blood Glucose Level	Befor:				Time:		
		After:				Time:		

SNACKS								
	Snack Totals							

Daily Totals							

Bedtime Blood Glucose Level		Time:	

Water	Sleep	Medication	Activity	Minutes	Notes

Notes

Diabetes Log Book

| Date: | | | | | M T W T F S S | | | |

	Meal	Cal	Fat	Carbs	Total Sugar	Added Sugar	Protein	Fiber
BREAKFAST								
	Breakfast Totals							
	Blood Glucose Level	Befor:			Time:			
		After:			Time:			

LUNCH								
	Lunch Totals							
	Blood Glucose Level	Befor:			Time:			
		After:			Time:			

DINNER								
	Dinner Totals							
	Blood Glucose Level	Befor:			Time:			
		After:			Time:			

SNACKS								
	Snack Totals							

Daily Totals							

Bedtime Blood Glucose Level		Time:	

Water	Sleep	Medication	Activity	Minutes	Notes

Diabetes Log Book

| Date: | | | | | | M T W T F S S | | | |

	Meal	Cal	Fat	Carbs	Total Sugar	Added Sugar	Protein	Fiber
BREAKFAST								
	Breakfast Totals							
	Blood Glucose Level	Befor:				Time:		
		After:				Time:		

LUNCH								
	Lunch Totals							
	Blood Glucose Level	Befor:				Time:		
		After:				Time:		

DINNER								
	Dinner Totals							
	Blood Glucose Level	Befor:				Time:		
		After:				Time:		

SNACKS								
	Snack Totals							

Daily Totals								

Bedtime Blood Glucose Level		Time:	

Water	Sleep	Medication	Activity	Minutes	Notes

Diabetes Log Book

Date:					M T W T F S S			

	Meal	Cal	Fat	Carbs	Total Sugar	Added Sugar	Protein	Fiber
BREAKFAST								
	Breakfast Totals							
	Blood Glucose Level	Befor:				Time:		
		After:				Time:		

LUNCH								
	Lunch Totals							
	Blood Glucose Level	Befor:				Time:		
		After:				Time:		

DINNER								
	DinnerTotals							
	Blood Glucose Level	Befor:				Time:		
		After:				Time:		

SNACKS								
	Snack Totals							

Daily Totals						

Bedtime Blood Glucose Level		Time:	

Water	Sleep	Medication	Activity	Minutes	Notes

Diabetes Log Book

Date:					M T W T F S S			

	Meal	Cal	Fat	Carbs	Total Sugar	Added Sugar	Protein	Fiber
BREAKFAST								
	Breakfast Totals							
	Blood Glucose Level	Befor:				Time:		
		After:				Time:		

		Cal	Fat	Carbs	Total Sugar	Added Sugar	Protein	Fiber
LUNCH								
	Lunch Totals							
	Blood Glucose Level	Befor:				Time:		
		After:				Time:		

		Cal	Fat	Carbs	Total Sugar	Added Sugar	Protein	Fiber
DINNER								
	Dinner Totals							
	Blood Glucose Level	Befor:				Time:		
		After:				Time:		

SNACKS								
	Snack Totals							

Daily Totals							

Bedtime Blood Glucose Level		Time:	

Water	Sleep	Medication	Activity	Minutes	Notes

Diabetes Log Book

| Date: | | | | | M | T | W | T | F | S | S |

	Meal	Cal	Fat	Carbs	Total Sugar	Added Sugar	Protein	Fiber
BREAKFAST								
	Breakfast Totals							
	Blood Glucose Level	Befor:				Time:		
		After:				Time:		

	Meal	Cal	Fat	Carbs	Total Sugar	Added Sugar	Protein	Fiber
LUNCH								
	Lunch Totals							
	Blood Glucose Level	Befor:				Time:		
		After:				Time:		

	Meal	Cal	Fat	Carbs	Total Sugar	Added Sugar	Protein	Fiber
DINNER								
	DinnerTotals							
	Blood Glucose Level	Befor:				Time:		
		After:				Time:		

SNACKS								
	Snack Totals							

Daily Totals							

Bedtime Blood Glucose Level		Time:	

Water	Sleep	Medication	Activity	Minutes	Notes

Notes

Diabetes Log Book

| Date: | | | | | M | T | W | T | F | S | S |

	Meal	Cal	Fat	Carbs	Total Sugar	Added Sugar	Protein	Fiber
BREAKFAST								
	Breakfast Totals							
	Blood Glucose Level	Befor:				Time:		
		After:				Time:		

	Meal							
LUNCH								
	Lunch Totals							
	Blood Glucose Level	Befor:				Time:		
		After:				Time:		

	Meal							
DINNER								
	Dinner Totals							
	Blood Glucose Level	Befor:				Time:		
		After:				Time:		

SNACKS								
	Snack Totals							

Daily Totals							

Bedtime Blood Glucose Level		Time:	

Water	Sleep	Medication	Activity	Minutes	Notes

Diabetes Log Book

| Date: | | | | | | | M | T | W | T | F | S | S |

	Meal	Cal	Fat	Carbs	Total Sugar	Added Sugar	Protein	Fiber
BREAKFAST								
	Breakfast Totals							
	Blood Glucose Level	Befor:				Time:		
		After:				Time:		

	Meal	Cal	Fat	Carbs	Total Sugar	Added Sugar	Protein	Fiber
LUNCH								
	Lunch Totals							
	Blood Glucose Level	Befor:				Time:		
		After:				Time:		

	Meal	Cal	Fat	Carbs	Total Sugar	Added Sugar	Protein	Fiber
DINNER								
	Dinner Totals							
	Blood Glucose Level	Befor:				Time:		
		After:				Time:		

		Cal	Fat	Carbs	Total Sugar	Added Sugar	Protein	Fiber
SNACKS								
	Snack Totals							

| Daily Totals | | | | | | | |

| Bedtime Blood Glucose Level | | Time: | |

Water	Sleep	Medication	Activity	Minutes	Notes

Diabetes Log Book

Date:					M T W T F S S			

	Meal	Cal	Fat	Carbs	Total Sugar	Added Sugar	Protein	Fiber
BREAKFAST								
	Breakfast Totals							
	Blood Glucose Level	Befor:				Time:		
		After:				Time:		

		Cal	Fat	Carbs	Total Sugar	Added Sugar	Protein	Fiber
LUNCH								
	Lunch Totals							
	Blood Glucose Level	Befor:				Time:		
		After:				Time:		

		Cal	Fat	Carbs	Total Sugar	Added Sugar	Protein	Fiber
DINNER								
	Dinner Totals							
	Blood Glucose Level	Befor:				Time:		
		After:				Time:		

SNACKS								
	Snack Totals							

Daily Totals							

Bedtime Blood Glucose Level		Time:	

Water	Sleep	Medication	Activity	Minutes	Notes

Diabetes Log Book

Date:						M	T	W	T	F	S	S

	Meal	Cal	Fat	Carbs	Total Sugar	Added Sugar	Protein	Fiber
BREAKFAST								
	Breakfast Totals							
	Blood Glucose Level	Befor:				Time:		
		After:				Time:		
LUNCH								
	Lunch Totals							
	Blood Glucose Level	Befor:				Time:		
		After:				Time:		
DINNER								
	Dinner Totals							
	Blood Glucose Level	Befor:				Time:		
		After:				Time:		
SNACKS								
	Snack Totals							
	Daily Totals							

Bedtime Blood Glucose Level		Time:	

Water	Sleep	Medication	Activity	Minutes	Notes

Diabetes Log Book

Date:				M T W T F S S			

	Meal	Cal	Fat	Carbs	Total Sugar	Added Sugar	Protein	Fiber
BREAKFAST								
	Breakfast Totals							
	Blood Glucose Level	Befor:			Time:			
		After:			Time:			

	Meal							
LUNCH								
	Lunch Totals							
	Blood Glucose Level	Befor:			Time:			
		After:			Time:			

	Meal							
DINNER								
	Dinner Totals							
	Blood Glucose Level	Befor:			Time:			
		After:			Time:			

	Meal							
SNACKS								
	Snack Totals							

Daily Totals							

Bedtime Blood Glucose Level		Time:	

Water	Sleep	Medication	Activity	Minutes	Notes

Diabetes Log Book

Date:							M T W T F S S		

	Meal	Cal	Fat	Carbs	Total Sugar	Added Sugar	Protein	Fiber
BREAKFAST								
	Breakfast Totals							
	Blood Glucose Level	Befor:				Time:		
		After:				Time:		

LUNCH								
	Lunch Totals							
	Blood Glucose Level	Befor:				Time:		
		After:				Time:		

DINNER								
	Dinner Totals							
	Blood Glucose Level	Befor:				Time:		
		After:				Time:		

SNACKS								
	Snack Totals							

	Daily Totals							

Bedtime Blood Glucose Level			Time:	

Water	Sleep	Medication	Activity	Minutes	Notes

Notes

Diabetes Log Book

| Date: | | | | | M T W T F S S | | | |

	Meal	Cal	Fat	Carbs	Total Sugar	Added Sugar	Protein	Fiber
BREAKFAST								
	Breakfast Totals							
	Blood Glucose Level	Befor:				Time:		
		After:				Time:		

LUNCH								
	Lunch Totals							
	Blood Glucose Level	Befor:				Time:		
		After:				Time:		

DINNER								
	Dinner Totals							
	Blood Glucose Level	Befor:				Time:		
		After:				Time:		

SNACKS								
	Snack Totals							

Daily Totals							

Bedtime Blood Glucose Level		Time:	

Water	Sleep	Medication	Activity	Minutes	Notes

Diabetes Log Book

| Date: | | | | M T W T F S S | | | | |

	Meal	Cal	Fat	Carbs	Total Sugar	Added Sugar	Protein	Fiber
BREAKFAST								
	Breakfast Totals							
	Blood Glucose Level	Befor:			Time:			
		After:			Time:			

		Cal	Fat	Carbs	Total Sugar	Added Sugar	Protein	Fiber
LUNCH								
	Lunch Totals							
	Blood Glucose Level	Befor:			Time:			
		After:			Time:			

		Cal	Fat	Carbs	Total Sugar	Added Sugar	Protein	Fiber
DINNER								
	DinnerTotals							
	Blood Glucose Level	Befor:			Time:			
		After:			Time:			

SNACKS								
	Snack Totals							

Daily Totals						

Bedtime Blood Glucose Level		Time:	

Water	Sleep	Medication	Activity	Minutes	Notes

Diabetes Log Book

| Date: | | | | | | M | T | W | T | F | S | S |

	Meal	Cal	Fat	Carbs	Total Sugar	Added Sugar	Protein	Fiber
BREAKFAST								
	Breakfast Totals							
	Blood Glucose Level	Befor:			Time:			
		After:			Time:			

		Cal	Fat	Carbs	Total Sugar	Added Sugar	Protein	Fiber
LUNCH								
	Lunch Totals							
	Blood Glucose Level	Befor:			Time:			
		After:			Time:			

		Cal	Fat	Carbs	Total Sugar	Added Sugar	Protein	Fiber
DINNER								
	Dinner Totals							
	Blood Glucose Level	Befor:			Time:			
		After:			Time:			

SNACKS								
	Snack Totals							

Daily Totals							

Bedtime Blood Glucose Level		Time:	

Water	Sleep	Medication	Activity	Minutes	Notes

Diabetes Log Book

| Date: | | | | | M T W T F S S | | | |

	Meal	Cal	Fat	Carbs	Total Sugar	Added Sugar	Protein	Fiber
BREAKFAST								
	Breakfast Totals							
	Blood Glucose Level	Befor:				Time:		
		After:				Time:		

LUNCH								
	Lunch Totals							
	Blood Glucose Level	Befor:				Time:		
		After:				Time:		

DINNER								
	Dinner Totals							
	Blood Glucose Level	Befor:				Time:		
		After:				Time:		

SNACKS								
	Snack Totals							

Daily Totals					

Bedtime Blood Glucose Level		Time:	

Water	Sleep	Medication	Activity	Minutes	Notes

Diabetes Log Book

Date:							M T W T F S S		

	Meal	Cal	Fat	Carbs	Total Sugar	Added Sugar	Protein	Fiber
BREAKFAST								
	Breakfast Totals							
	Blood Glucose Level	Befor:				Time:		
		After:				Time:		

LUNCH								
	Lunch Totals							
	Blood Glucose Level	Befor:				Time:		
		After:				Time:		

DINNER								
	Dinner Totals							
	Blood Glucose Level	Befor:				Time:		
		After:				Time:		

SNACKS							
	Snack Totals						

Daily Totals							

Bedtime Blood Glucose Level		Time:	

Water	Sleep	Medication	Activity	Minutes	Notes

Notes

Diabetes Log Book

Date:						M	T	W	T	F	S	S

BREAKFAST	Meal	Cal	Fat	Carbs	Total Sugar	Added Sugar	Protein	Fiber
	Breakfast Totals							
	Blood Glucose Level	Befor:			Time:			
		After:			Time:			

LUNCH								
	Lunch Totals							
	Blood Glucose Level	Befor:			Time:			
		After:			Time:			

DINNER								
	Dinner Totals							
	Blood Glucose Level	Befor:			Time:			
		After:			Time:			

SNACKS								
	Snack Totals							

Daily Totals							

Bedtime Blood Glucose Level		Time:

Water	Sleep	Medication	Activity	Minutes	Notes

Diabetes Log Book

| Date: | | | | | M T W T F S S | | | |

	Meal	Cal	Fat	Carbs	Total Sugar	Added Sugar	Protein	Fiber
BREAKFAST								
	Breakfast Totals							
	Blood Glucose Level	Befor:				Time:		
		After:				Time:		

LUNCH								
	Lunch Totals							
	Blood Glucose Level	Befor:				Time:		
		After:				Time:		

DINNER								
	Dinner Totals							
	Blood Glucose Level	Befor:				Time:		
		After:				Time:		

SNACKS								
	Snack Totals							

Daily Totals						

Bedtime Blood Glucose Level		Time:	

Water	Sleep	Medication	Activity	Minutes	Notes

Diabetes Log Book

Date:						M T W T F S S		

	Meal	Cal	Fat	Carbs	Total Sugar	Added Sugar	Protein	Fiber
BREAKFAST								
	Breakfast Totals							
	Blood Glucose Level	Befor:				Time:		
		After:				Time:		

LUNCH								
	Lunch Totals							
	Blood Glucose Level	Befor:				Time:		
		After:				Time:		

DINNER								
	DinnerTotals							
	Blood Glucose Level	Befor:				Time:		
		After:				Time:		

SNACKS								
	Snack Totals							

Daily Totals								

Bedtime Blood Glucose Level		Time:

Water	Sleep	Medication	Activity	Minutes	Notes

Diabetes Log Book

Date:				M	T	W	T	F	S	S

	Meal	Cal	Fat	Carbs	Total Sugar	Added Sugar	Protein	Fiber
BREAKFAST								
	Breakfast Totals							
	Blood Glucose Level	Befor:				Time:		
		After:				Time:		
LUNCH								
	Lunch Totals							
	Blood Glucose Level	Befor:				Time:		
		After:				Time:		
DINNER								
	Dinner Totals							
	Blood Glucose Level	Befor:				Time:		
		After:				Time:		
SNACKS								
	Snack Totals							
	Daily Totals							

Bedtime Blood Glucose Level		Time:	

Water	Sleep	Medication	Activity	Minutes	Notes

Diabetes Log Book

Date:					M T W T F S S			

	Meal	Cal	Fat	Carbs	Total Sugar	Added Sugar	Protein	Fiber
BREAKFAST								
	Breakfast Totals							
	Blood Glucose Level	Befor:				Time:		
		After:				Time:		

	Meal	Cal	Fat	Carbs	Total Sugar	Added Sugar	Protein	Fiber
LUNCH								
	Lunch Totals							
	Blood Glucose Level	Befor:				Time:		
		After:				Time:		

	Meal	Cal	Fat	Carbs	Total Sugar	Added Sugar	Protein	Fiber
DINNER								
	Dinner Totals							
	Blood Glucose Level	Befor:				Time:		
		After:				Time:		

SNACKS								
	Snack Totals							

Daily Totals							

Bedtime Blood Glucose Level		Time:	

Water	Sleep	Medication	Activity	Minutes	Notes

Diabetes Log Book

Date:					M T W T F S S			

	Meal	Cal	Fat	Carbs	Total Sugar	Added Sugar	Protein	Fiber
BREAKFAST								
	Breakfast Totals							
	Blood Glucose Level	Befor:				Time:		
		After:				Time:		

	Meal	Cal	Fat	Carbs	Total Sugar	Added Sugar	Protein	Fiber
LUNCH								
	Lunch Totals							
	Blood Glucose Level	Befor:				Time:		
		After:				Time:		

	Meal	Cal	Fat	Carbs	Total Sugar	Added Sugar	Protein	Fiber
DINNER								
	Dinner Totals							
	Blood Glucose Level	Befor:				Time:		
		After:				Time:		

SNACKS								
	Snack Totals							

Daily Totals							

Bedtime Blood Glucose Level		Time:	

Water	Sleep	Medication	Activity	Minutes	Notes

Notes

Diabetes Log Book

| Date: | | | | | M | T | W | T | F | S | S |

	Meal	Cal	Fat	Carbs	Total Sugar	Added Sugar	Protein	Fiber
BREAKFAST								
	Breakfast Totals							
	Blood Glucose Level	Befor:				Time:		
		After:				Time:		

		Cal	Fat	Carbs	Total Sugar	Added Sugar	Protein	Fiber
LUNCH								
	Lunch Totals							
	Blood Glucose Level	Befor:				Time:		
		After:				Time:		

		Cal	Fat	Carbs	Total Sugar	Added Sugar	Protein	Fiber
DINNER								
	DinnerTotals							
	Blood Glucose Level	Befor:				Time:		
		After:				Time:		

SNACKS								
	Snack Totals							

Daily Totals							

Bedtime Blood Glucose Level		Time:	

Water	Sleep	Medication	Activity	Minutes	Notes

Diabetes Log Book

Date:						M T W T F S S		

	Meal	Cal	Fat	Carbs	Total Sugar	Added Sugar	Protein	Fiber
BREAKFAST								
	Breakfast Totals							
	Blood Glucose Level	Befor:				Time:		
		After:				Time:		

LUNCH								
	Lunch Totals							
	Blood Glucose Level	Befor:				Time:		
		After:				Time:		

DINNER								
	Dinner Totals							
	Blood Glucose Level	Befor:				Time:		
		After:				Time:		

SNACKS								
	Snack Totals							

Daily Totals							

Bedtime Blood Glucose Level		Time:

Water	Sleep	Medication	Activity	Minutes	Notes

Diabetes Log Book

| Date: | | | | | M | T | W | T | F | S | S |

	Meal	Cal	Fat	Carbs	Total Sugar	Added Sugar	Protein	Fiber
BREAKFAST								
	Breakfast Totals							
	Blood Glucose Level	Befor:				Time:		
		After:				Time:		

	Meal	Cal	Fat	Carbs	Total Sugar	Added Sugar	Protein	Fiber
LUNCH								
	Lunch Totals							
	Blood Glucose Level	Befor:				Time:		
		After:				Time:		

	Meal	Cal	Fat	Carbs	Total Sugar	Added Sugar	Protein	Fiber
DINNER								
	Dinner Totals							
	Blood Glucose Level	Befor:				Time:		
		After:				Time:		

SNACKS								
	Snack Totals							

Daily Totals							

Bedtime Blood Glucose Level		Time:	

Water	Sleep	Medication	Activity	Minutes	Notes

Diabetes Log Book

Date:	M T W T F S S

	Meal	Cal	Fat	Carbs	Total Sugar	Added Sugar	Protein	Fiber
BREAKFAST								
	Breakfast Totals							
	Blood Glucose Level	Befor:				Time:		
		After:				Time:		

LUNCH								
	Lunch Totals							
	Blood Glucose Level	Befor:				Time:		
		After:				Time:		

DINNER								
	Dinner Totals							
	Blood Glucose Level	Befor:				Time:		
		After:				Time:		

SNACKS								
	Snack Totals							

Daily Totals							

Bedtime Blood Glucose Level		Time:	

Water	Sleep	Medication	Activity	Minutes	Notes

Diabetes Log Book

| Date: | | | | | M | T | W | T | F | S | S |

	Meal	Cal	Fat	Carbs	Total Sugar	Added Sugar	Protein	Fiber
BREAKFAST								
	Breakfast Totals							
	Blood Glucose Level	Befor:				Time:		
		After:				Time:		

LUNCH								
	Lunch Totals							
	Blood Glucose Level	Befor:				Time:		
		After:				Time:		

DINNER								
	DinnerTotals							
	Blood Glucose Level	Befor:				Time:		
		After:				Time:		

SNACKS								
	Snack Totals							

| Daily Totals | | | | | | |

| Bedtime Blood Glucose Level | | Time: | |

Water	Sleep	Medication	Activity	Minutes	Notes

Notes

Diabetes Log Book

Date:				M T W T F S S			

BREAKFAST

Meal	Cal	Fat	Carbs	Total Sugar	Added Sugar	Protein	Fiber
Breakfast Totals							
Blood Glucose Level	Befor:			Time:			
	After:			Time:			

LUNCH

Lunch Totals							
Blood Glucose Level	Befor:			Time:			
	After:			Time:			

DINNER

Dinner Totals							
Blood Glucose Level	Befor:			Time:			
	After:			Time:			

SNACKS

Snack Totals							

Daily Totals							

Bedtime Blood Glucose Level		Time:	

Water	Sleep	Medication	Activity	Minutes	Notes

Diabetes Log Book

Date:						M	T	W	T	F	S	S

	Meal	Cal	Fat	Carbs	Total Sugar	Added Sugar	Protein	Fiber
BREAKFAST								
	Breakfast Totals							
	Blood Glucose Level	Befor:				Time:		
		After:				Time:		
LUNCH								
	Lunch Totals							
	Blood Glucose Level	Befor:				Time:		
		After:				Time:		
DINNER								
	Dinner Totals							
	Blood Glucose Level	Befor:				Time:		
		After:				Time:		
SNACKS								
	Snack Totals							
	Daily Totals							

Bedtime Blood Glucose Level		Time:

Water	Sleep	Medication	Activity	Minutes	Notes

Diabetes Log Book

Date:					M T W T F S S			

Meal	Cal	Fat	Carbs	Total Sugar	Added Sugar	Protein	Fiber
BREAKFAST							
Breakfast Totals							
Blood Glucose Level — Befor:				Time:			
After:				Time:			

LUNCH							
Lunch Totals							
Blood Glucose Level — Befor:				Time:			
After:				Time:			

DINNER							
Dinner Totals							
Blood Glucose Level — Befor:				Time:			
After:				Time:			

SNACKS							
Snack Totals							

Daily Totals							

Bedtime Blood Glucose Level		Time:	

Water	Sleep	Medication	Activity	Minutes	Notes

Diabetes Log Book

Date:					M T W T F S S			

	Meal	Cal	Fat	Carbs	Total Sugar	Added Sugar	Protein	Fiber
BREAKFAST								
	Breakfast Totals							
	Blood Glucose Level	Befor:				Time:		
		After:				Time:		

LUNCH								
	Lunch Totals							
	Blood Glucose Level	Befor:				Time:		
		After:				Time:		

DINNER								
	Dinner Totals							
	Blood Glucose Level	Befor:				Time:		
		After:				Time:		

SNACKS								
	Snack Totals							

Daily Totals								

Bedtime Blood Glucose Level		Time:	

Water	Sleep	Medication	Activity	Minutes	Notes

Diabetes Log Book

| Date: | | | | M | T | W | T | F | S | S |

	Meal	Cal	Fat	Carbs	Total Sugar	Added Sugar	Protein	Fiber
BREAKFAST								
	Breakfast Totals							
	Blood Glucose Level	Befor:				Time:		
		After:				Time:		

	Meal	Cal	Fat	Carbs	Total Sugar	Added Sugar	Protein	Fiber
LUNCH								
	Lunch Totals							
	Blood Glucose Level	Befor:				Time:		
		After:				Time:		

	Meal	Cal	Fat	Carbs	Total Sugar	Added Sugar	Protein	Fiber
DINNER								
	DinnerTotals							
	Blood Glucose Level	Befor:				Time:		
		After:				Time:		

		Cal	Fat	Carbs	Total Sugar	Added Sugar	Protein	Fiber
SNACKS								
	Snack Totals							

| Daily Totals | | | | | | | |

| Bedtime Blood Glucose Level | | Time: | |

Water	Sleep	Medication	Activity	Minutes	Notes

Notes

Diabetes Log Book

Date:					M	T	W	T	F	S	S

	Meal	Cal	Fat	Carbs	Total Sugar	Added Sugar	Protein	Fiber
BREAKFAST								
	Breakfast Totals							
	Blood Glucose Level	Befor:			Time:			
		After:			Time:			

		Cal	Fat	Carbs	Total Sugar	Added Sugar	Protein	Fiber
LUNCH								
	Lunch Totals							
	Blood Glucose Level	Befor:			Time:			
		After:			Time:			

		Cal	Fat	Carbs	Total Sugar	Added Sugar	Protein	Fiber
DINNER								
	DinnerTotals							
	Blood Glucose Level	Befor:			Time:			
		After:			Time:			

SNACKS								
	Snack Totals							

Daily Totals							

Bedtime Blood Glucose Level		Time:	

Water	Sleep	Medication	Activity	Minutes	Notes

Diabetes Log Book

| Date: | | | | | | | M | T | W | T | F | S | S |

	Meal	Cal	Fat	Carbs	Total Sugar	Added Sugar	Protein	Fiber
BREAKFAST								
	Breakfast Totals							
	Blood Glucose Level	Befor:				Time:		
		After:				Time:		

		Cal	Fat	Carbs	Total Sugar	Added Sugar	Protein	Fiber
LUNCH								
	Lunch Totals							
	Blood Glucose Level	Befor:				Time:		
		After:				Time:		

		Cal	Fat	Carbs	Total Sugar	Added Sugar	Protein	Fiber
DINNER								
	Dinner Totals							
	Blood Glucose Level	Befor:				Time:		
		After:				Time:		

SNACKS								
	Snack Totals							

	Daily Totals							

Bedtime Blood Glucose Level		Time:	

Water	Sleep	Medication	Activity	Minutes	Notes

Diabetes Log Book

| Date: | | | | | M T W T F S S | | | |

BREAKFAST	Meal	Cal	Fat	Carbs	Total Sugar	Added Sugar	Protein	Fiber
	Breakfast Totals							
	Blood Glucose Level	Befor:				Time:		
		After:				Time:		

LUNCH	Meal	Cal	Fat	Carbs	Total Sugar	Added Sugar	Protein	Fiber
	Lunch Totals							
	Blood Glucose Level	Befor:				Time:		
		After:				Time:		

DINNER	Meal	Cal	Fat	Carbs	Total Sugar	Added Sugar	Protein	Fiber
	Dinner Totals							
	Blood Glucose Level	Befor:				Time:		
		After:				Time:		

SNACKS								
	Snack Totals							

Daily Totals							

Bedtime Blood Glucose Level		Time:

Water	Sleep	Medication	Activity	Minutes	Notes

Diabetes Log Book

Date:						M	T	W	T	F	S	S

	Meal	Cal	Fat	Carbs	Total Sugar	Added Sugar	Protein	Fiber
BREAKFAST								
	Breakfast Totals							
	Blood Glucose Level	Befor:				Time:		
		After:				Time:		
LUNCH								
	Lunch Totals							
	Blood Glucose Level	Befor:				Time:		
		After:				Time:		
DINNER								
	Dinner Totals							
	Blood Glucose Level	Befor:				Time:		
		After:				Time:		
SNACKS								
	Snack Totals							
	Daily Totals							

Bedtime Blood Glucose Level		Time:

Water	Sleep	Medication	Activity	Minutes	Notes

Diabetes Log Book

| Date: | | | | | M | T | W | T | F | S | S |

	Meal	Cal	Fat	Carbs	Total Sugar	Added Sugar	Protein	Fiber
BREAKFAST								
	Breakfast Totals							
	Blood Glucose Level	Befor:				Time:		
		After:				Time:		

LUNCH								
	Lunch Totals							
	Blood Glucose Level	Befor:				Time:		
		After:				Time:		

DINNER								
	Dinner Totals							
	Blood Glucose Level	Befor:				Time:		
		After:				Time:		

SNACKS								
	Snack Totals							

Daily Totals							

Bedtime Blood Glucose Level		Time:

Water	Sleep	Medication	Activity	Minutes	Notes

Notes

Diabetes Log Book

Date:					M T W T F S S			

BREAKFAST

Meal	Cal	Fat	Carbs	Total Sugar	Added Sugar	Protein	Fiber
Breakfast Totals							
Blood Glucose Level	Befor:			Time:			
	After:			Time:			

LUNCH

Lunch Totals							
Blood Glucose Level	Befor:			Time:			
	After:			Time:			

DINNER

Dinner Totals							
Blood Glucose Level	Befor:			Time:			
	After:			Time:			

SNACKS

Snack Totals							

Daily Totals							

Bedtime Blood Glucose Level		Time:	

Water	Sleep	Medication	Activity	Minutes	Notes

Diabetes Log Book

Date:							M T W T F S S		

	Meal	Cal	Fat	Carbs	Total Sugar	Added Sugar	Protein	Fiber
BREAKFAST								
	Breakfast Totals							
	Blood Glucose Level	Befor:				Time:		
		After:				Time:		

	Meal	Cal	Fat	Carbs	Total Sugar	Added Sugar	Protein	Fiber
LUNCH								
	Lunch Totals							
	Blood Glucose Level	Befor:				Time:		
		After:				Time:		

	Meal	Cal	Fat	Carbs	Total Sugar	Added Sugar	Protein	Fiber
DINNER								
	Dinner Totals							
	Blood Glucose Level	Befor:				Time:		
		After:				Time:		

SNACKS								
	Snack Totals							

Daily Totals							

Bedtime Blood Glucose Level		Time:	

Water	Sleep	Medication	Activity	Minutes	Notes

Diabetes Log Book

Date:					M	T	W	T	F	S	S

	Meal	Cal	Fat	Carbs	Total Sugar	Added Sugar	Protein	Fiber
BREAKFAST								
	Breakfast Totals							
	Blood Glucose Level	Befor:				Time:		
		After:				Time:		

LUNCH								
	Lunch Totals							
	Blood Glucose Level	Befor:				Time:		
		After:				Time:		

DINNER								
	Dinner Totals							
	Blood Glucose Level	Befor:				Time:		
		After:				Time:		

SNACKS								
	Snack Totals							

Daily Totals							

Bedtime Blood Glucose Level		Time:	

Water	Sleep	Medication	Activity	Minutes	Notes

Diabetes Log Book

| Date: | | | | | | M T W T F S S | | | |

	Meal	Cal	Fat	Carbs	Total Sugar	Added Sugar	Protein	Fiber
BREAKFAST								
	Breakfast Totals							
	Blood Glucose Level	Befor:				Time:		
		After:				Time:		

LUNCH								
	Lunch Totals							
	Blood Glucose Level	Befor:				Time:		
		After:				Time:		

DINNER								
	Dinner Totals							
	Blood Glucose Level	Befor:				Time:		
		After:				Time:		

SNACKS								
	Snack Totals							

Daily Totals							

Bedtime Blood Glucose Level		Time:	

Water	Sleep	Medication	Activity	Minutes	Notes

Diabetes Log Book

Date:				M	T	W	T	F	S	S

	Meal	Cal	Fat	Carbs	Total Sugar	Added Sugar	Protein	Fiber
BREAKFAST								
	Breakfast Totals							
	Blood Glucose Level	Befor:				Time:		
		After:				Time:		
LUNCH								
	Lunch Totals							
	Blood Glucose Level	Befor:				Time:		
		After:				Time:		
DINNER								
	Dinner Totals							
	Blood Glucose Level	Befor:				Time:		
		After:				Time:		
SNACKS								
	Snack Totals							
	Daily Totals							

Bedtime Blood Glucose Level		Time:

Water	Sleep	Medication	Activity	Minutes	Notes

Notes

Diabetes Log Book

Date:					M	T	W	T	F	S	S

	Meal	Cal	Fat	Carbs	Total Sugar	Added Sugar	Protein	Fiber
BREAKFAST								
	Breakfast Totals							
	Blood Glucose Level	Befor:			Time:			
		After:			Time:			

LUNCH								
	Lunch Totals							
	Blood Glucose Level	Befor:			Time:			
		After:			Time:			

DINNER								
	Dinner Totals							
	Blood Glucose Level	Befor:			Time:			
		After:			Time:			

SNACKS								
	Snack Totals							

Daily Totals							

Bedtime Blood Glucose Level		Time:	

Water	Sleep	Medication	Activity	Minutes	Notes

Diabetes Log Book

Date:						M T W T F S S		

	Meal	Cal	Fat	Carbs	Total Sugar	Added Sugar	Protein	Fiber
BREAKFAST								
	Breakfast Totals							
	Blood Glucose Level	Befor:				Time:		
		After:				Time:		

LUNCH								
	Lunch Totals							
	Blood Glucose Level	Befor:				Time:		
		After:				Time:		

DINNER								
	Dinner Totals							
	Blood Glucose Level	Befor:				Time:		
		After:				Time:		

SNACKS								
	Snack Totals							

Daily Totals							

Bedtime Blood Glucose Level		Time:	

Water	Sleep	Medication	Activity	Minutes	Notes

Diabetes Log Book

Date:					M	T	W	T	F	S	S

	Meal	Cal	Fat	Carbs	Total Sugar	Added Sugar	Protein	Fiber
BREAKFAST								
	Breakfast Totals							
	Blood Glucose Level	Befor:				Time:		
		After:				Time:		

LUNCH								
	Lunch Totals							
	Blood Glucose Level	Befor:				Time:		
		After:				Time:		

DINNER								
	Dinner Totals							
	Blood Glucose Level	Befor:				Time:		
		After:				Time:		

SNACKS								
	Snack Totals							

	Daily Totals							

Bedtime Blood Glucose Level		Time:	

Water	Sleep	Medication	Activity	Minutes	Notes

Diabetes Log Book

Date:					M T W T F S S			

	Meal	Cal	Fat	Carbs	Total Sugar	Added Sugar	Protein	Fiber
BREAKFAST								
	Breakfast Totals							
	Blood Glucose Level	Befor:			Time:			
		After:			Time:			

LUNCH								
	Lunch Totals							
	Blood Glucose Level	Befor:			Time:			
		After:			Time:			

DINNER								
	Dinner Totals							
	Blood Glucose Level	Befor:			Time:			
		After:			Time:			

SNACKS								
	Snack Totals							

Daily Totals							

Bedtime Blood Glucose Level		Time:	

Water	Sleep	Medication	Activity	Minutes	Notes

Diabetes Log Book

| Date: | | | | | M T W T F S S | | | |

	Meal	Cal	Fat	Carbs	Total Sugar	Added Sugar	Protein	Fiber
BREAKFAST								
	Breakfast Totals							
	Blood Glucose Level	Befor:				Time:		
		After:				Time:		

	Meal							
LUNCH								
	Lunch Totals							
	Blood Glucose Level	Befor:				Time:		
		After:				Time:		

	Meal							
DINNER								
	Dinner Totals							
	Blood Glucose Level	Befor:				Time:		
		After:				Time:		

SNACKS								
	Snack Totals							

Daily Totals							

Bedtime Blood Glucose Level		Time:	

Water	Sleep	Medication	Activity	Minutes	Notes

Notes

Diabetes Log Book

Date:					M T W T F S S			

	Meal	Cal	Fat	Carbs	Total Sugar	Added Sugar	Protein	Fiber
BREAKFAST								
	Breakfast Totals							
	Blood Glucose Level	Befor:				Time:		
		After:				Time:		

LUNCH								
	Lunch Totals							
	Blood Glucose Level	Befor:				Time:		
		After:				Time:		

DINNER								
	Dinner Totals							
	Blood Glucose Level	Befor:				Time:		
		After:				Time:		

SNACKS								
	Snack Totals							

Daily Totals								

Bedtime Blood Glucose Level		Time:	

Water	Sleep	Medication	Activity	Minutes	Notes

Diabetes Log Book

| Date: | | | | | | M | T | W | T | F | S | S |

	Meal	Cal	Fat	Carbs	Total Sugar	Added Sugar	Protein	Fiber
BREAKFAST								
	Breakfast Totals							
	Blood Glucose Level	Befor:				Time:		
		After:				Time:		

LUNCH								
	Lunch Totals							
	Blood Glucose Level	Befor:				Time:		
		After:				Time:		

DINNER								
	Dinner Totals							
	Blood Glucose Level	Befor:				Time:		
		After:				Time:		

SNACKS								
	Snack Totals							

Daily Totals							

Bedtime Blood Glucose Level		Time:

Water	Sleep	Medication	Activity	Minutes	Notes

Diabetes Log Book

| Date: | | | | | | M | T | W | T | F | S | S |

	Meal	Cal	Fat	Carbs	Total Sugar	Added Sugar	Protein	Fiber
BREAKFAST								
	Breakfast Totals							
	Blood Glucose Level	Befor:				Time:		
		After:				Time:		

		Cal	Fat	Carbs	Total Sugar	Added Sugar	Protein	Fiber
LUNCH								
	Lunch Totals							
	Blood Glucose Level	Befor:				Time:		
		After:				Time:		

		Cal	Fat	Carbs	Total Sugar	Added Sugar	Protein	Fiber
DINNER								
	Dinner Totals							
	Blood Glucose Level	Befor:				Time:		
		After:				Time:		

SNACKS								
	Snack Totals							

Daily Totals							

Bedtime Blood Glucose Level		Time:	

Water	Sleep	Medication	Activity	Minutes	Notes

Diabetes Log Book

Date:						M T W T F S S			

	Meal	Cal	Fat	Carbs	Total Sugar	Added Sugar	Protein	Fiber
BREAKFAST								
	Breakfast Totals							
	Blood Glucose Level	Befor:				Time:		
		After:				Time:		

	Meal	Cal	Fat	Carbs	Total Sugar	Added Sugar	Protein	Fiber
LUNCH								
	Lunch Totals							
	Blood Glucose Level	Befor:				Time:		
		After:				Time:		

	Meal	Cal	Fat	Carbs	Total Sugar	Added Sugar	Protein	Fiber
DINNER								
	Dinner Totals							
	Blood Glucose Level	Befor:				Time:		
		After:				Time:		

SNACKS								
	Snack Totals							

Daily Totals							

Bedtime Blood Glucose Level		Time:	

Water	Sleep	Medication	Activity	Minutes	Notes

Diabetes Log Book

Date:					M	T	W	T	F	S	S

	Meal	Cal	Fat	Carbs	Total Sugar	Added Sugar	Protein	Fiber
BREAKFAST								
	Breakfast Totals							
	Blood Glucose Level	Befor:			Time:			
		After:			Time:			

LUNCH								
	Lunch Totals							
	Blood Glucose Level	Befor:			Time:			
		After:			Time:			

DINNER								
	Dinner Totals							
	Blood Glucose Level	Befor:			Time:			
		After:			Time:			

SNACKS								
	Snack Totals							

Daily Totals							

Bedtime Blood Glucose Level		Time:	

Water	Sleep	Medication	Activity	Minutes	Notes

Notes

Diabetes Log Book

Date:						M T W T F S S			

	Meal	Cal	Fat	Carbs	Total Sugar	Added Sugar	Protein	Fiber
BREAKFAST								
	Breakfast Totals							
	Blood Glucose Level	Befor:			Time:			
		After:			Time:			

		Cal	Fat	Carbs	Total Sugar	Added Sugar	Protein	Fiber
LUNCH								
	Lunch Totals							
	Blood Glucose Level	Befor:			Time:			
		After:			Time:			

		Cal	Fat	Carbs	Total Sugar	Added Sugar	Protein	Fiber
DINNER								
	Dinner Totals							
	Blood Glucose Level	Befor:			Time:			
		After:			Time:			

SNACKS								
	Snack Totals							

Daily Totals							

Bedtime Blood Glucose Level		Time:	

Water	Sleep	Medication	Activity	Minutes	Notes

Diabetes Log Book

| Date: | | | | | M | T | W | T | F | S | S |

	Meal	Cal	Fat	Carbs	Total Sugar	Added Sugar	Protein	Fiber
BREAKFAST								
	Breakfast Totals							
	Blood Glucose Level	Befor:				Time:		
		After:				Time:		

		Cal	Fat	Carbs	Total Sugar	Added Sugar	Protein	Fiber
LUNCH								
	Lunch Totals							
	Blood Glucose Level	Befor:				Time:		
		After:				Time:		

		Cal	Fat	Carbs	Total Sugar	Added Sugar	Protein	Fiber
DINNER								
	Dinner Totals							
	Blood Glucose Level	Befor:				Time:		
		After:				Time:		

SNACKS								
	Snack Totals							

| Daily Totals | | | | | | | |

| Bedtime Blood Glucose Level | | Time: | |

Water	Sleep	Medication	Activity	Minutes	Notes

Diabetes Log Book

Date:					M	T	W	T	F	S	S

	Meal	Cal	Fat	Carbs	Total Sugar	Added Sugar	Protein	Fiber
BREAKFAST								
	Breakfast Totals							
	Blood Glucose Level	Befor:				Time:		
		After:				Time:		

		Cal	Fat	Carbs	Total Sugar	Added Sugar	Protein	Fiber
LUNCH								
	Lunch Totals							
	Blood Glucose Level	Befor:				Time:		
		After:				Time:		

		Cal	Fat	Carbs	Total Sugar	Added Sugar	Protein	Fiber
DINNER								
	Dinner Totals							
	Blood Glucose Level	Befor:				Time:		
		After:				Time:		

SNACKS								
	Snack Totals							

Daily Totals							

Bedtime Blood Glucose Level		Time:	

Water	Sleep	Medication	Activity	Minutes	Notes

Diabetes Log Book

Date:						M T W T F S S		

	Meal	Cal	Fat	Carbs	Total Sugar	Added Sugar	Protein	Fiber
BREAKFAST								
	Breakfast Totals							
	Blood Glucose Level	Befor:				Time:		
		After:				Time:		

LUNCH								
	Lunch Totals							
	Blood Glucose Level	Befor:				Time:		
		After:				Time:		

DINNER								
	Dinner Totals							
	Blood Glucose Level	Befor:				Time:		
		After:				Time:		

SNACKS								
	Snack Totals							

Daily Totals							

Bedtime Blood Glucose Level		Time:	

Water	Sleep	Medication	Activity	Minutes	Notes

Diabetes Log Book

| Date: | | | | | | M | T | W | T | F | S | S |

<table>
<tr><td rowspan="7">BREAKFAST</td><td>Meal</td><td>Cal</td><td>Fat</td><td>Carbs</td><td>Total Sugar</td><td>Added Sugar</td><td>Protein</td><td>Fiber</td></tr>
<tr><td></td><td></td><td></td><td></td><td></td><td></td><td></td><td></td></tr>
<tr><td></td><td></td><td></td><td></td><td></td><td></td><td></td><td></td></tr>
<tr><td></td><td></td><td></td><td></td><td></td><td></td><td></td><td></td></tr>
<tr><td>Breakfast Totals</td><td></td><td></td><td></td><td></td><td></td><td></td><td></td></tr>
<tr><td rowspan="2">Blood Glucose Level</td><td colspan="2">Befor:</td><td colspan="3">Time:</td><td colspan="2"></td></tr>
<tr><td colspan="2">After:</td><td colspan="3">Time:</td><td colspan="2"></td></tr>
</table>

<table>
<tr><td rowspan="5">LUNCH</td><td></td><td></td><td></td><td></td><td></td><td></td><td></td><td></td></tr>
<tr><td></td><td></td><td></td><td></td><td></td><td></td><td></td><td></td></tr>
<tr><td>Lunch Totals</td><td></td><td></td><td></td><td></td><td></td><td></td><td></td></tr>
<tr><td rowspan="2">Blood Glucose Level</td><td colspan="2">Befor:</td><td colspan="3">Time:</td><td colspan="2"></td></tr>
<tr><td colspan="2">After:</td><td colspan="3">Time:</td><td colspan="2"></td></tr>
</table>

<table>
<tr><td rowspan="5">DINNER</td><td></td><td></td><td></td><td></td><td></td><td></td><td></td><td></td></tr>
<tr><td></td><td></td><td></td><td></td><td></td><td></td><td></td><td></td></tr>
<tr><td>Dinner Totals</td><td></td><td></td><td></td><td></td><td></td><td></td><td></td></tr>
<tr><td rowspan="2">Blood Glucose Level</td><td colspan="2">Befor:</td><td colspan="3">Time:</td><td colspan="2"></td></tr>
<tr><td colspan="2">After:</td><td colspan="3">Time:</td><td colspan="2"></td></tr>
</table>

<table>
<tr><td rowspan="3">SNACKS</td><td></td><td></td><td></td><td></td><td></td><td></td><td></td><td></td></tr>
<tr><td></td><td></td><td></td><td></td><td></td><td></td><td></td><td></td></tr>
<tr><td>Snack Totals</td><td></td><td></td><td></td><td></td><td></td><td></td><td></td></tr>
</table>

Daily Totals							

Bedtime Blood Glucose Level		Time:

Water	Sleep	Medication	Activity	Minutes	Notes

Diabetes Log Book

Date:						M	T	W	T	F	S	S

	Meal	Cal	Fat	Carbs	Total Sugar	Added Sugar	Protein	Fiber
BREAKFAST								
	Breakfast Totals							
	Blood Glucose Level	Befor:				Time:		
		After:				Time:		
LUNCH								
	Lunch Totals							
	Blood Glucose Level	Befor:				Time:		
		After:				Time:		
DINNER								
	Dinner Totals							
	Blood Glucose Level	Befor:				Time:		
		After:				Time:		
SNACKS								
	Snack Totals							
	Daily Totals							

Bedtime Blood Glucose Level		Time:

Water	Sleep	Medication	Activity	Minutes	Notes

Notes

Diabetes Log Book

| Date: | | | | | M T W T F S S | | | | |

	Meal	Cal	Fat	Carbs	Total Sugar	Added Sugar	Protein	Fiber
BREAKFAST								
	Breakfast Totals							
	Blood Glucose Level	Befor:				Time:		
		After:				Time:		

	Meal							
LUNCH								
	Lunch Totals							
	Blood Glucose Level	Befor:				Time:		
		After:				Time:		

	Meal							
DINNER								
	Dinner Totals							
	Blood Glucose Level	Befor:				Time:		
		After:				Time:		

SNACKS								
	Snack Totals							

Daily Totals							

Bedtime Blood Glucose Level		Time:	

Water	Sleep	Medication	Activity	Minutes	Notes

Diabetes Log Book

| Date: | | | | | M | T | W | T | F | S | S |

	Meal	Cal	Fat	Carbs	Total Sugar	Added Sugar	Protein	Fiber
BREAKFAST								
	Breakfast Totals							
	Blood Glucose Level	Befor:				Time:		
		After:				Time:		

	Meal	Cal	Fat	Carbs	Total Sugar	Added Sugar	Protein	Fiber
LUNCH								
	Lunch Totals							
	Blood Glucose Level	Befor:				Time:		
		After:				Time:		

	Meal	Cal	Fat	Carbs	Total Sugar	Added Sugar	Protein	Fiber
DINNER								
	Dinner Totals							
	Blood Glucose Level	Befor:				Time:		
		After:				Time:		

SNACKS								
	Snack Totals							

Daily Totals							

Bedtime Blood Glucose Level		Time:	

Water	Sleep	Medication	Activity	Minutes	Notes

Diabetes Log Book

Date:						M T W T F S S			

	Meal	Cal	Fat	Carbs	Total Sugar	Added Sugar	Protein	Fiber
BREAKFAST								
	Breakfast Totals							
	Blood Glucose Level	Befor:				Time:		
		After:				Time:		
LUNCH								
	Lunch Totals							
	Blood Glucose Level	Befor:				Time:		
		After:				Time:		
DINNER								
	Dinner Totals							
	Blood Glucose Level	Befor:				Time:		
		After:				Time:		
SNACKS								
	Snack Totals							

	Daily Totals							

Bedtime Blood Glucose Level		Time:	

Water	Sleep	Medication	Activity	Minutes	Notes

Diabetes Log Book

| Date: | | | | | M | T | W | T | F | S | S |

	Meal	Cal	Fat	Carbs	Total Sugar	Added Sugar	Protein	Fiber
BREAKFAST								
	Breakfast Totals							
	Blood Glucose Level	Befor:				Time:		
		After:				Time:		

	Meal	Cal	Fat	Carbs	Total Sugar	Added Sugar	Protein	Fiber
LUNCH								
	Lunch Totals							
	Blood Glucose Level	Befor:				Time:		
		After:				Time:		

	Meal	Cal	Fat	Carbs	Total Sugar	Added Sugar	Protein	Fiber
DINNER								
	Dinner Totals							
	Blood Glucose Level	Befor:				Time:		
		After:				Time:		

SNACKS								
	Snack Totals							

Daily Totals							

Bedtime Blood Glucose Level		Time:	

Water	Sleep	Medication	Activity	Minutes	Notes

Diabetes Log Book

Date:					M T W T F S S			

	Meal	Cal	Fat	Carbs	Total Sugar	Added Sugar	Protein	Fiber
BREAKFAST								
	Breakfast Totals							
	Blood Glucose Level	Befor:				Time:		
		After:				Time:		
LUNCH								
	Lunch Totals							
	Blood Glucose Level	Befor:				Time:		
		After:				Time:		
DINNER								
	Dinner Totals							
	Blood Glucose Level	Befor:				Time:		
		After:				Time:		
SNACKS								
	Snack Totals							
	Daily Totals							

Bedtime Blood Glucose Level		Time:	

Water	Sleep	Medication	Activity	Minutes	Notes

Notes

Diabetes Log Book

| Date: | | | | | | M | T | W | T | F | S | S |

	Meal	Cal	Fat	Carbs	Total Sugar	Added Sugar	Protein	Fiber
BREAKFAST								
	Breakfast Totals							
	Blood Glucose Level	Befor:				Time:		
		After:				Time:		
LUNCH								
	Lunch Totals							
	Blood Glucose Level	Befor:				Time:		
		After:				Time:		
DINNER								
	Dinner Totals							
	Blood Glucose Level	Befor:				Time:		
		After:				Time:		
SNACKS								
	Snack Totals							
	Daily Totals							

| Bedtime Blood Glucose Level | | Time: | |

Water	Sleep	Medication	Activity	Minutes	Notes

Diabetes Log Book

Date:					M	T	W	T	F	S	S

BREAKFAST

Meal	Cal	Fat	Carbs	Total Sugar	Added Sugar	Protein	Fiber
Breakfast Totals							
Blood Glucose Level	Befor:			Time:			
	After:			Time:			

LUNCH

Meal							
Lunch Totals							
Blood Glucose Level	Befor:			Time:			
	After:			Time:			

DINNER

Meal							
Dinner Totals							
Blood Glucose Level	Befor:			Time:			
	After:			Time:			

SNACKS

Meal							
Snack Totals							

Daily Totals							

Bedtime Blood Glucose Level		Time:	

Water	Sleep	Medication	Activity	Minutes	Notes

Diabetes Log Book

| Date: | | | | | M T W T F S S | | | |

	Meal	Cal	Fat	Carbs	Total Sugar	Added Sugar	Protein	Fiber
BREAKFAST								
	Breakfast Totals							
	Blood Glucose Level	Befor:				Time:		
		After:				Time:		

	Meal	Cal	Fat	Carbs	Total Sugar	Added Sugar	Protein	Fiber
LUNCH								
	Lunch Totals							
	Blood Glucose Level	Befor:				Time:		
		After:				Time:		

	Meal	Cal	Fat	Carbs	Total Sugar	Added Sugar	Protein	Fiber
DINNER								
	Dinner Totals							
	Blood Glucose Level	Befor:				Time:		
		After:				Time:		

SNACKS								
	Snack Totals							

Daily Totals							

Bedtime Blood Glucose Level		Time:	

Water	Sleep	Medication	Activity	Minutes	Notes

Diabetes Log Book

Date:					M T W T F S S			

	Meal	Cal	Fat	Carbs	Total Sugar	Added Sugar	Protein	Fiber
BREAKFAST								
	Breakfast Totals							
	Blood Glucose Level	Befor:				Time:		
		After:				Time:		

LUNCH								
	Lunch Totals							
	Blood Glucose Level	Befor:				Time:		
		After:				Time:		

DINNER								
	Dinner Totals							
	Blood Glucose Level	Befor:				Time:		
		After:				Time:		

SNACKS								
	Snack Totals							

Daily Totals							

Bedtime Blood Glucose Level		Time:	

Water	Sleep	Medication	Activity	Minutes	Notes

Notes

Diabetes Log Book

Date:						M	T	W	T	F	S	S

Meal	Cal	Fat	Carbs	Total Sugar	Added Sugar	Protein	Fiber
BREAKFAST							
Breakfast Totals							
Blood Glucose Level — Befor:			Time:				
After:			Time:				
LUNCH							
Lunch Totals							
Blood Glucose Level — Befor:			Time:				
After:			Time:				
DINNER							
Dinner Totals							
Blood Glucose Level — Befor:			Time:				
After:			Time:				
SNACKS							
Snack Totals							
Daily Totals							

Bedtime Blood Glucose Level		Time:	

Water	Sleep	Medication	Activity	Minutes	Notes

Diabetes Log Book

Date:					M T W T F S S			

	Meal	Cal	Fat	Carbs	Total Sugar	Added Sugar	Protein	Fiber
BREAKFAST								
	Breakfast Totals							
	Blood Glucose Level	Befor:				Time:		
		After:				Time:		

	Meal							
LUNCH								
	Lunch Totals							
	Blood Glucose Level	Befor:				Time:		
		After:				Time:		

	Meal							
DINNER								
	Dinner Totals							
	Blood Glucose Level	Befor:				Time:		
		After:				Time:		

SNACKS								
	Snack Totals							

Daily Totals							

Bedtime Blood Glucose Level		Time:	

Water	Sleep	Medication	Activity	Minutes	Notes

Diabetes Log Book

| Date: | | | | | | M | T | W | T | F | S | S |

	Meal	Cal	Fat	Carbs	Total Sugar	Added Sugar	Protein	Fiber
BREAKFAST								
	Breakfast Totals							
	Blood Glucose Level	Befor:			Time:			
		After:			Time:			

LUNCH								
	Lunch Totals							
	Blood Glucose Level	Befor:			Time:			
		After:			Time:			

DINNER								
	DinnerTotals							
	Blood Glucose Level	Befor:			Time:			
		After:			Time:			

SNACKS								
	Snack Totals							

Daily Totals							

Bedtime Blood Glucose Level		Time:	

Water	Sleep	Medication	Activity	Minutes	Notes

Diabetes Log Book

| Date: | | | | | | M | T | W | T | F | S | S |

	Meal	Cal	Fat	Carbs	Total Sugar	Added Sugar	Protein	Fiber
BREAKFAST								
	Breakfast Totals							
	Blood Glucose Level	Befor:				Time:		
		After:				Time:		

LUNCH								
	Lunch Totals							
	Blood Glucose Level	Befor:				Time:		
		After:				Time:		

DINNER								
	Dinner Totals							
	Blood Glucose Level	Befor:				Time:		
		After:				Time:		

SNACKS								
	Snack Totals							

Daily Totals							

Bedtime Blood Glucose Level		Time:	

Water	Sleep	Medication	Activity	Minutes	Notes

Diabetes Log Book

Date:				M	T	W	T	F	S	S

	Meal	Cal	Fat	Carbs	Total Sugar	Added Sugar	Protein	Fiber
BREAKFAST								
	Breakfast Totals							
	Blood Glucose Level	Befor:				Time:		
		After:				Time:		

LUNCH								
	Lunch Totals							
	Blood Glucose Level	Befor:				Time:		
		After:				Time:		

DINNER								
	Dinner Totals							
	Blood Glucose Level	Befor:				Time:		
		After:				Time:		

SNACKS								
	Snack Totals							

Daily Totals							

Bedtime Blood Glucose Level		Time:	

Water	Sleep	Medication	Activity	Minutes	Notes

Diabetes Log Book

| Date: | | | | | | | | M | T | W | T | F | S | S |

	Meal	Cal	Fat	Carbs	Total Sugar	Added Sugar	Protein	Fiber
BREAKFAST								
	Breakfast Totals							
	Blood Glucose Level	Befor:				Time:		
		After:				Time:		

	Meal	Cal	Fat	Carbs	Total Sugar	Added Sugar	Protein	Fiber
LUNCH								
	Lunch Totals							
	Blood Glucose Level	Befor:				Time:		
		After:				Time:		

	Meal	Cal	Fat	Carbs	Total Sugar	Added Sugar	Protein	Fiber
DINNER								
	Dinner Totals							
	Blood Glucose Level	Befor:				Time:		
		After:				Time:		

SNACKS								
	Snack Totals							

Daily Totals							

Bedtime Blood Glucose Level		Time:	

Water	Sleep	Medication	Activity	Minutes	Notes

Diabetes Log Book

| Date: | | | | M | T | W | T | F | S | S |

	Meal	Cal	Fat	Carbs	Total Sugar	Added Sugar	Protein	Fiber
BREAKFAST								
	Breakfast Totals							
	Blood Glucose Level	Befor:			Time:			
		After:			Time:			

	Meal	Cal	Fat	Carbs	Total Sugar	Added Sugar	Protein	Fiber
LUNCH								
	Lunch Totals							
	Blood Glucose Level	Befor:			Time:			
		After:			Time:			

	Meal	Cal	Fat	Carbs	Total Sugar	Added Sugar	Protein	Fiber
DINNER								
	Dinner Totals							
	Blood Glucose Level	Befor:			Time:			
		After:			Time:			

SNACKS								
	Snack Totals							

| Daily Totals | | | | | | | |

| Bedtime Blood Glucose Level | | Time: | |

Water	Sleep	Medication	Activity	Minutes	Notes

Diabetes Log Book

Date:					M	T	W	T	F	S	S

	Meal	Cal	Fat	Carbs	Total Sugar	Added Sugar	Protein	Fiber
BREAKFAST								
	Breakfast Totals							
	Blood Glucose Level	Befor:				Time:		
		After:				Time:		
LUNCH								
	Lunch Totals							
	Blood Glucose Level	Befor:				Time:		
		After:				Time:		
DINNER								
	Dinner Totals							
	Blood Glucose Level	Befor:				Time:		
		After:				Time:		
SNACKS								
	Snack Totals							
	Daily Totals							

Bedtime Blood Glucose Level		Time:	

Water	Sleep	Medication	Activity	Minutes	Notes

Diabetes Log Book

Date:					M	T	W	T	F	S	S

	Meal	Cal	Fat	Carbs	Total Sugar	Added Sugar	Protein	Fiber
BREAKFAST								
	Breakfast Totals							
	Blood Glucose Level	Befor:				Time:		
		After:				Time:		

LUNCH								
	Lunch Totals							
	Blood Glucose Level	Befor:				Time:		
		After:				Time:		

DINNER								
	Dinner Totals							
	Blood Glucose Level	Befor:				Time:		
		After:				Time:		

SNACKS								
	Snack Totals							

Daily Totals							

Bedtime Blood Glucose Level		Time:

Water	Sleep	Medication	Activity	Minutes	Notes

Diabetes Log Book

| Date: | | | | | | | M | T | W | T | F | S | S |

	Meal	Cal	Fat	Carbs	Total Sugar	Added Sugar	Protein	Fiber
BREAKFAST								
	Breakfast Totals							
	Blood Glucose Level	Befor:				Time:		
		After:				Time:		

	Meal	Cal	Fat	Carbs	Total Sugar	Added Sugar	Protein	Fiber
LUNCH								
	Lunch Totals							
	Blood Glucose Level	Befor:				Time:		
		After:				Time:		

	Meal	Cal	Fat	Carbs	Total Sugar	Added Sugar	Protein	Fiber
DINNER								
	Dinner Totals							
	Blood Glucose Level	Befor:				Time:		
		After:				Time:		

SNACKS								
	Snack Totals							

Daily Totals							

Bedtime Blood Glucose Level		Time:	

Water	Sleep	Medication	Activity	Minutes	Notes

Notes

Diabetes Log Book

| Date: | | | | | | M T W T F S S | | | |

	Meal	Cal	Fat	Carbs	Total Sugar	Added Sugar	Protein	Fiber
BREAKFAST								
	Breakfast Totals							
	Blood Glucose Level	Befor:				Time:		
		After:				Time:		

LUNCH								
	Lunch Totals							
	Blood Glucose Level	Befor:				Time:		
		After:				Time:		

DINNER								
	Dinner Totals							
	Blood Glucose Level	Befor:				Time:		
		After:				Time:		

SNACKS								
	Snack Totals							

Daily Totals							

Bedtime Blood Glucose Level		Time:

Water	Sleep	Medication	Activity	Minutes	Notes

Diabetes Log Book

Date:				M T W T F S S

	Meal	Cal	Fat	Carbs	Total Sugar	Added Sugar	Protein	Fiber
BREAKFAST								
	Breakfast Totals							
	Blood Glucose Level	Befor:			Time:			
		After:			Time:			

	Meal	Cal	Fat	Carbs	Total Sugar	Added Sugar	Protein	Fiber
LUNCH								
	Lunch Totals							
	Blood Glucose Level	Befor:			Time:			
		After:			Time:			

	Meal	Cal	Fat	Carbs	Total Sugar	Added Sugar	Protein	Fiber
DINNER								
	DinnerTotals							
	Blood Glucose Level	Befor:			Time:			
		After:			Time:			

SNACKS								
	Snack Totals							

Daily Totals							

Bedtime Blood Glucose Level		Time:	

Water	Sleep	Medication	Activity	Minutes	Notes

Diabetes Log Book

| Date: | | | | | | M T W T F S S | | | |

	Meal	Cal	Fat	Carbs	Total Sugar	Added Sugar	Protein	Fiber
BREAKFAST								
	Breakfast Totals							
	Blood Glucose Level	Befor:				Time:		
		After:				Time:		

LUNCH								
	Lunch Totals							
	Blood Glucose Level	Befor:				Time:		
		After:				Time:		

DINNER								
	Dinner Totals							
	Blood Glucose Level	Befor:				Time:		
		After:				Time:		

SNACKS								
	Snack Totals							

Daily Totals							

Bedtime Blood Glucose Level		Time:	

Water	Sleep	Medication	Activity	Minutes	Notes

Diabetes Log Book

| Date: | | | | | M | T | W | T | F | S | S |

	Meal	Cal	Fat	Carbs	Total Sugar	Added Sugar	Protein	Fiber
BREAKFAST								
	Breakfast Totals							
	Blood Glucose Level	Befor:				Time:		
		After:				Time:		

		Cal	Fat	Carbs	Total Sugar	Added Sugar	Protein	Fiber
LUNCH								
	Lunch Totals							
	Blood Glucose Level	Befor:				Time:		
		After:				Time:		

		Cal	Fat	Carbs	Total Sugar	Added Sugar	Protein	Fiber
DINNER								
	Dinner Totals							
	Blood Glucose Level	Befor:				Time:		
		After:				Time:		

SNACKS								
	Snack Totals							

| Daily Totals | | | | | | | |

| Bedtime Blood Glucose Level | | Time: | |

Water	Sleep	Medication	Activity	Minutes	Notes

Notes

Thank you!

WE ARE GLAD THAT YOU PURCHASED OUR
BOOK!
PLEASE LET US KNOW HOW WE CAN IMPROVE IT!
YOUR FEEDBACK IS ESSENTIAL TO US.

Contact us at:

M   log'Sin@gmail.com

JUST TITLE THE EMAIL 'CREATIVE' AND WE WILL

GIVE YOU SOME EXTRA SURPRISES!